Guide to

HERITAGE ASSESSMENT
AND HEALTH TRADITIONS

Guide to HERITAGE ASSESSMENT AND HEALTH TRADITIONS

Rachel E. Spector, PhD, RN, CTN, FAAN
Associate Professor
Boston College School of Nursing
Chestnut Hill, Massachusetts

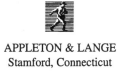

APPLETON & LANGE
Stamford, Connecticut

Copyright © 1996 by Appleton & Lange
A Simon & Schuster Company

All rights reserved. This book, or any parts thereof, may not be used or
reproduced in any manner without written permission. For information,
address Appleton & Lange, P.O. Box 120041, Stamford, Connecticut
06902-0041.

96 97 98 99 / 10 9 8 7 6 5 4 3 2 1

Prentice Hall International (UK) Limited, *London*
Prentice Hall of Australia Pty. Limited, *Sydney*
Prentice Hall Canada, Inc., *Toronto*
Prentice Hall Hispanoamericana, S.A., *Mexico*
Prentice Hall of India Private Limited, *New Delhi*
Prentice Hall of Japan, Inc., *Tokyo*
Simon & Schuster Asia Pte. Ltd., *Singapore*
Editora Prentice Hall do Brasil Ltda., *Rio de Janeiro*
Prentice Hall, *Upper Saddle River, New Jersey*

ISBN 0-8385-1484-7

9 780838 514849 90000

Editor-in-Chief: Sally J. Barhydt
Production Editor: Sondra Greenfield
Designer: Janice Barsevich Bielawa

PRINTED IN THE UNITED STATES OF AMERICA

Contents

Introduction 1

Heritage Assessment Tool 2

Cultural Phenomena Affecting Health 6

Health Traditions Assessment Model 11

Health Traditions Assessment Guidelines 13

Community Traditions Assessment Guidelines 16

Selected Health Traditions 20

Cross-Cultural Health-Care Guide 33

Sample Grids for Cultural Health Assessment 35

Introduction

....

This guide presents a selection of practical assessment tools, guidelines, and information, the purpose of which is to facilitate communication and caring for the culturally diverse people you will meet in all practice arenas. Each of us comes from a unique cultural heritage, and the health-care system in which we practice may present us with complex cultural dilemmas. As you begin to delve into this topic, apply the tools to yourself and then ask the following questions about your personal and professional worlds:

- What is my personal ethnocultural heritage and how deeply do I identify with it?
- What do I know about holistic health and illness from my own heritage?
- What is my professional heritage and how deeply do I identify with it?
- What have I learned about holistic health and illness in the contexts of both my professional heritage and the health-care delivery system?

1

Heritage Assessment Tool

This set of questions can be used to investigate a given client's or your own ethnic, cultural, and religious heritage. It can help you to perform a heritage assessment to determine how deeply a given person identifies with a particular *tradition*. It is most useful in setting the stage for understanding a person's health traditions. The greater the number of positive responses, the greater the person's identification with a traditional heritage. The one exception to positive answers is the question about family name change. This question may be answered negatively.

1. Where was your mother born? _____

2. Where was your father born? _____

3. Where were your grandparents born?

   a. Your mother's mother? _____

   b. Your mother's father? _____

   c. Your father's mother? _____

   d. Your father's father? _____

4. How many brothers _____ and sisters _____ do you have?

5. What setting did you grow up in? Urban _____ Rural _____ Suburban _____

6. What country did your parents grow up in?

   Father _____

   Mother _____

7. How old were you when you came to the United States? _____

8. How old were your parents when they came to the United States?

   Mother _____

   Father _____

9. When you were growing up, who lived with you?

   _____

10. Have you maintained contact with

    a. Aunts, uncles, cousins? (1) Yes _____ (2) No _____

    b. Brothers and sisters? (1) Yes _____ (2) No _____

    c. Parents? (1) Yes _____ (2) No _____

    d. Your own children? (1) Yes _____ (2) No _____

11. Did most of your aunts, uncles, cousins live near your home?

    (1) Yes _____ (2) No _____

12. Approximately how often did you visit your family members who lived outside your home?

    (1) Daily _____ (2) Weekly _____ (3) Monthly _____

    (4) Once a year or less _____ (5) Never _____

13. Was your original family name changed?

    (1) Yes _____ (2) No _____

14. What is your religious preference?

    (1) Catholic _____ (2) Jewish _____

    (3) Protestant _____ Denomination _____

    (4) Other _____ (5) None _____

15. Is your spouse the same religion as you?

    (1) Yes _____ (2) No _____

16. Is your spouse the same ethnic background as you?

    (1) Yes _____   (2) No _____

17. What kind of school did you go to?

    (1) Public _____   (2) Private _____   (3) Parochial _____

18. As an adult, do you live in a neighborhood where the neighbors are the same religion and ethnic background as yourself?

    (1) Yes _____   (2) No _____

19. Do you belong to a religious institution?

    (1) Yes _____   (2) No _____

20. Would you describe yourself as an active member?

    (1) Yes _____   (2) No _____

21. How often do you attend your religious institution?

    (1) More than once a week _____   (2) Weekly _____
    (3) Monthly _____   (4) Special holidays only _____
    (5) Never _____

22. Do you practice your religion in your home?

    (1) Yes _____   (2) No _____   (if yes, please specify)
    (3) Praying _____   (4) Bible reading _____
    (5) Diet _____   (6) Celebrating religious holidays _____

23. Do you prepare foods of your ethnic background?

    (1) Yes _____   (2) No _____

24. Do you participate in ethnic activities?

    (1) Yes _____   (2) No _____   (if yes, please specify)
    (3) Singing _____   (4) Holiday celebrations _____
    (5) Dancing _____   (6) Festivals _____
    (7) Costumes _____   (8) Other _____

25. Are your friends from the same religious background as you?

    (1) Yes _____   (2) No _____

26. Are your friends from the same ethnic background as you?

    (1) Yes _____   (2) No _____

27. What is your native language? _____

28. Do you speak this language?

    (1) Prefer _____   (2) Occasionally _____   (3) Rarely _____

29. Do you read your native language?

    (1) Yes _____   (2) No _____

Cultural Phenomena Affecting Health

Giger and Davidhizar* have identified six cultural phenomena that vary among cultural groups. These are

1. **Environmental control**—The ability of members of a particular cultural group to plan activities that control nature or direct environmental factors. Included are the complex systems of traditional health and illness beliefs, the practice of folk medicine, and the use of traditional healers. These play an extremely important role in the way clients respond to health-related experiences, including the ways in which they define health and illness and seek and use health-care resources and social supports.
2. **Biological variations**—People from one cultural group differ biologically (physically and genetically) from members of other cultural groups:
   a. Body build and structure
   b. Skin color
   c. Enzymatic and genetic variations
   d. Susceptibility to disease
   e. Nutritional variations

---

*Giger, J.N. and Davidhizar, R.E. *Transcultural Nursing Assessment and Intervention, 2nd ed.* St. Louis: Mosby, 1995, pp. 19, 43, 61, 89, 113, and 127.

3. **Social organization**—The family unit, (nuclear, single-parent, or extended family) and the social group organizations (religious or ethnic) with which clients and families may identify.
4. **Communication**—Communication differences are presented in many ways, including language differences, verbal and nonverbal behaviors, and silence.
5. **Space**—Personal space and territoriality involves people's behaviors and attitudes toward the space around themselves and are influenced by culture. The following terms indicate different types of space and relate to acceptable behaviors within these zones:
   a. *Intimate zone:* extends up to 1½ feet.
   b. *Personal distance:* extends from 1½ to 4 feet.
   c. *Social distance:* extends from 4 to 12 feet.
   d. *Public distance:* extends 12 feet or more.
6. **Time Orientation**—The viewing of the time in the present, past, or future varies among different cultural groups.
   a. *Future-oriented*—People are concerned with long-range goals and with health-care measures taken in the present to prevent the occurrence of illness in the future.
   b. *Present-oriented*—People are oriented more to the present than the future and may be late for appointments because they are less concerned about planning ahead to be on time.

CULTURAL PHENOMENA AFFECTING HEALTH CARE

	African (Black) Americans	Asian/Pacific Islander Americans	American Indians Aleuts, and Eskimos	Hispanic Americans	European (White) Origin Americans
Nations of Origin:	West coast (as slaves) of Africa Many African countries West Indian islands Dominican Republic Haiti Jamaica	China, Japan, Hawaii, the Philippines, Vietnam, Asian India, Korea, Samoa, Guam, and the remaining Asian/Pacific islands	200 American Indian nations indigenous to North America Aleuts, and Eskimos in Alaska	Hispanic countries Spain, Cuba, Mexico, Central and South America Puerto Rico	Germany, England, Italy, Ireland, Former Soviet Union, and all other European countries
Environmental Control:	Traditional health and illness beliefs may continue to be observed by "traditional" people	Traditional health and illness beliefs may continued to be observed by "traditional" people	Traditional health and illness beliefs may continue to be observed by "traditional" people Natural and magicoreligious folk medicine tradition Traditional healer: medicine man or woman	Traditional health and illness beliefs may continue to be observed by "traditional" people Folk medicine tradition Traditional healers: *curandero, espiritista, partera, señora*	Primary reliance on "modern," Western" health-care delivery system Remaining traditional health and illness beliefs and practices may be observed Some remaining traditional folk medicine Homeopathic medicine resurgent

8

EXAMPLES OF CULTURAL PHENOMENA AFFECTING HEALTH CARE (CONT.)

	African (Black) Americans (cont.)	Asian/Pacific Islander Americans (cont.)	American Indians Aleuts, and Eskimos (cont.)	Hispanic Americans (cont.)	European (White) Origin Americans (cont.)
Biological Variations:	Sickle cell anemia Hypertension Cancer of the esophagus Stomach cancer Coccidioidomycosis Lactose intolerance	Hypertension Liver cancer Stomach cancer Coccidioidomycosis Lactose intolerance Thalassemia	Accidents Heart disease Cirrhosis of the liver Diabetes mellitus	Diabetes mellitus Parasites Coccidioidomycosis Lactose intolerance	Breast cancer Heart disease Diabetes mellitus Thalassemia
Social Organization:	Family: many single-parent female-headed households Large, extended family networks Strong church affiliations within community Community social organizations	Family: hierarchical structure, loyalty Large, extended family networks Devotion to tradition Many religions, including Taoism, Buddhism, Islam, and Christianity Community social organizations	Extremely family-oriented to both biological and extended families Children are taught to respect traditions Community social organizations	Nuclear families Large, extended family networks *Compadrazzo* (godparents) Strong church affiliations within community Community social organizations	Nuclear families Extended families Judeo-Christian religions Community and social organizations

9

EXAMPLES OF CULTURAL PHENOMENA AFFECTING HEALTH CARE (CONT.)

	African (Black) Americans (cont.)	Asian/Pacific Islander Americans (cont.)	American Indians Aleuts, and Eskimos (cont.)	Hispanic Americans (cont.)	European (White) Origin Americans (cont.)
Communication:	National languages Dialect: Pidgin French, Spanish, Creole	National language preference Dialects, written characters Use of silence Nonverbal and contextual cueing	Tribal languages Use of silence and body language	Spanish or Portuguese are the primary languages	National languages Many learned English rapidly as immigrants Verbal, rather than nonverbal
Space:	Close personal space	Noncontact people	Space very important and has no boundaries	Tactile relationships: touch, handshakes, embrace Value physical presence	Noncontact people: aloof, distant Southern countries: closer contact and touch
Time Orientation:	Present over future	Present	Present	Present	Future over present

Adapted from: Spector, R. "Cultures, Ethnicity, and Nursing," in *Fundamentals of Nursing* (3rd ed.), eds. Potter, P. and Perry, A. (St. Louis: Mosby, 1992), p. 101.

Health Traditions Assessment Model

People who identify with a traditional ethnocultural heritage may tend to define health and illness in a holistic way, and have health beliefs and practices that differ from those of the Western, or modern, health-care delivery system.

Imagine holistic health as a three-dimensional phenomenon that encompasses the following: body (the physical self), mind (feelings, attitudes, and behavior), and spirit (the I who I am).

Health, in the traditional sense, is the state of balance within the body, mind, and spirit, and with the family, community, and the forces of the natural world.

Illness, is the opposite.

Many traditional health-related beliefs and practices exist today among people who know and live by the traditions of their given ethnocultural heritage.

Health, in this traditional context, has three dimensions each of which has three aspects, making a total of nine interrelated facets.

1. **Maintaining health**
    a. *Physical*—Are there special clothes one must wear; foods one must eat, not eat, or combinations to avoid; exercises one must do?

    b. *Mental*—Are there special sources of entertainment; games or other ways of concentrating; traditional "rules of behavior?"

    c. *Spiritual*—Are there special religious customs; prayers; meditations?

2. **Protecting health and preventing illness**

    a. *Physical*—Are there special foods that must be eaten after certain life events, such as childbirth; dietary taboos that must be adhered to; symbolic clothes that must be worn?

    b. *Mental*—Are there special people who must be avoided; rituals for self-protection; familial roles?

    c. *Spiritual*—Are there special religious customs; superstitions; amulets; oils or waters?

3. **Restoring health**

    a. *Physical*—Are there special folk remedies; liniments; procedures, such as cupping, acupuncture, and moxibustion?

    b. *Mental*—Are there special healers, such as *curanderos*, available; rituals; folk medicines?

    c. *Spiritual*—Are there special rituals and prayers; meditations; healers?

Traditional methods of maintaining health, protecting health and preventing illness, and restoring health require the knowledge and understanding of health-related resources from within a given person's ethnoreligious cultural heritage and community. These methods may be used instead of or along with modern methods of health care. They are not alternative methods of health care in the sense that they are methods that are an integral part of a person's given heritage.

Health Traditions Assessment Guidelines

A given client's interrelated health traditions can be assessed in countless ways. The following grids contain suggested questions and are parallel to the nine interrelated facets of health (the physical, mental, and spiritual aspects of the personal and communal dimensions of maintaining, protecting (preventing illness), and restoring health) that are a theme throughout *Cultural Diversity in Health and Illness* and this assessment guide.

ASSESSMENT GUIDE FOR *PERSONAL* METHODS TO MAINTAIN, PROTECT (PREVENT ILLNESS), AND RESTORE HEALTH

	Physical	Mental	Spiritual
Maintain Health	Are there special clothes you must wear at certain times of the day, week, year? Are there special foods you must eat at certain times? Do you have any dietary restrictions? Are there any foods that you cannot eat?	What do you do for activities, such as reading, sports, games? Do you have hobbies? Do you visit family often? Do you visit friends often?	Do you practice your religion and attend church or other communal activities? Do you pray or meditate? Do you observe religious customs? Do you belong to fraternal organizations?
Protect Health or Prevent Illness	Are there foods that you cannot eat together? Are there special foods that you must eat? Are there any types of clothing that you are not allowed to wear?	Are there people or situations that you have been taught to avoid? Do you take extraordinary precautions under certain circumstances? Do you take time for yourself?	Do you observe religious customs? Do you wear any amulets or hang them in your home? Do you have any practices, such as always opening the window when you sleep? Do you have any other practices to protect yourself from "harm"?

ASSESSMENT GUIDE FOR *PERSONAL* METHODS TO MAINTAIN, PROTECT (PREVENT ILLNESS), AND RESTORE HEALTH (CONT.)

	Physical (cont.)	Mental (cont.)	Spiritual (cont.)
Restore Health	What kinds of medicines do you take before you see a doctor or nurse? Are there herbs that you take? Are there special treatments that you use?	Do you know of any specific practices your mother or grandmother may use to relax? Do you know how big problems can be cared for in your community? Do you drink special teas to help you unwind or relax? Do you know of any healers?	Do you know of any religious rituals that help to restore health? Do you meditate? Did you ever go to a healing service? Do you know about exorcism?

Community Traditions Assessment Guidelines

Health traditions come alive the moment one leaves institutional confines and goes into the community. An indepth community assessment of an ethnoreligious community alerts you to the vast resources that exist within traditional communities and that may be tapped. The following outline serves as a community assessment guide:

Demographic data
- Total population size of entire city or town
- Breakdown by areas—residential concentrations
- Breakdown by ages
- Other breakdowns
    - Education
    - Occupations
    - Income
- Nations of origin of residents of the location and the target neighborhood

Traditional health and illness beliefs
- Definition of health
- Definition of illness
- Overall health status

Causes of illness
- Poor eating habits

- Wrong food combinations
- Viruses, bacteria, other organisms
- Punishment from God
- The evil eye
- Hexes, spells, or envy
- Witchcraft
- Environmental changes
- Exposure to drafts
- Over or underwork
- Grief and loss

Methods of maintaining health

Methods of protecting health and preventing illness

Methods of restoring health—home remedies

Visits and use of M.D. or other health-care resources

Health-care resources, such as neighborhood health centers

Anyone else within community who looks after people, such as traditional healers

Child-bearing beliefs and practices

Child-rearing beliefs and practices

Rituals and beliefs surrounding death and dying

Walk through the community and observe the traditional grocery stores, pharmacies, markets, jewelry stores, beauty parlors, morticians, and churches. If possible, visit several places, purchase remedies, eat in a restaurant, and observe services in a church.

ASSESSMENT GUIDE FOR *COMMUNAL* METHODS AND RESOURCES FOR MAINTAINING, PROTECTING (PREVENT ILLNESS), AND RESTORING HEALTH

	Physical	Mental	Spiritual
Maintain Health	Where are people able to purchase special clothing? Where are specific foods purchased? What types of health education are a part of the person's culture and who teaches this information? Where is the information obtained?	What are examples of culture-specific books, games, and other activities for this given client? Where are books, games, and other forms of culture-specific materials obtained? What are culture-specific rules for this client, such as conversation, eye contact?	Are there resources to meet the client's identified spiritual needs? How are the people and places accessed?
Protect Health or Prevent Illness	Where are special clothes obtained? What are some examples of symbolic clothing a person may obtain?	Who within the client's family and community teaches the cultural rules? Are there rules about avoiding people or places? Are there special activities that must be observed?	Who teaches the spiritual practices? Where can the client purchase special amulets and other symbolic objects? Are they costly? Are they readily available?

18

ASSESSMENT GUIDE FOR *COMMUNAL* METHODS AND RESOURCES FOR MAINTAINING, PROTECTING (PREVENT ILLNESS), AND RESTORING HEALTH (CONT.)

	Physical (cont.)	Mental (cont.)	Spiritual (cont.)
Restore Health	Where are various remedies purchased? Are people able to grow herbs and other remedies in their own homes? Where are other traditional services obtained? Who are the traditional healers within the person's community and where do they practice?	Who are the traditional people within the community that the person may seek care and advice from? Are there culture-specific activities, such as story telling that may be available to the client? Where are the ingredients for special "teas" purchased?	Are there traditional healers in the community? Who are they and how are they accessed?

SELECTED HEALTH TRADITIONS

Nation	Maintain Health	Protect Health or Prevent Illness	Restore Health
Austria	Soups and sleeping. Dress warmly and wear shoes.	Use "Schweden-bitter" (herb extract). Promote sweating.	Chest cold: Scoop inside of a bla... radish, fill the cavity with rock candy and bake it. Then drink the contents. Ear aches: Take a white sock and put heated salt inside of it and place it on the ear. Fever: Wrap wet towel around body. Cough: Melt sugar and crystallize with onion juice.
Bangladesh	Eat fruits and rice.	Eat a special plant from the rain forest.	Use herbs.
Bolivia	Sleep, eat, and drink in moderation.	Walk.	Use cupping to improve circulation.
Brazil	Take *Cachaca.* Cook and clean all day.	Drink herbal teas. Eat chicken soup.	Drink herbal teas. Eat herbs.
China	Always clean the floor. Use the Chinese herbs.	Drink ginger tea to prevent the flu.	Cough: Scratch the back with a coin. Drink herbal teas. Diarrhea: Drink a burned rice tea.

SELECTED HEALTH TRADITIONS (CONT.)

Nation (cont.)	Maintain Health (cont.)	Protect Health or Prevent Illness (cont.)	Restore Health (cont.)
Colombia	Drink *agua de panela con limon*. Eat garlic for general health. Eat chicken and rice.	Use *botanica* (herbal plants).	Cold: Prepare onions and oil by cooking until pulp is soft, strain, and eat with honey. Baby's colic: Prepare star anise tea. Nerves: Drink *tilo*. Cramps: Cook onion and place on stomach. Visit traditional healers.
Croatia	Eat organically grown food, goat's milk, fish from the Adriatic Sea.	Get plenty of fresh air and exercise.	Broken bones: Place a dead animal on the skin. Upset stomach: Drink chamomile tea. Earaches: Place hot oil on cotton ball in the ear.

SELECTED HEALTH TRADITIONS (CONT.)

Nation (cont.)	Maintain Health (cont.)	Protect Health or Prevent Illness (cont.)	Restore Health (cont.)
Cuba	Drink carrot juice and eat fruits, vegetables, garlic, tea soups, and stews.	Dress warmly.	Sore throat: Drink olive oil and salt, or a tea of boiled water with lemon rind for 10 minutes then put in cup with regular tea bag and juice of lemon, add honey to sweeten. Use pig skins as bandages to cure cuts. Visit traditional healers (*santero*).
Dominican Republic	Use oils or herb teas.	Keep the sick inside the house. Get a lot of rest. Keep out of cold rain.	Use plants, oils, and roots for homemade medicines. Cover a person with a fever with a heavy blanket for two to three hours until he or she sweats.
Ecuador	Eat healthy food; drink teas.	Drink teas. Wear amulets.	Drink teas.

SELECTED HEALTH TRADITIONS (CONT.)

Nation (cont.)	Maintain Health (cont.)	Protect Health or Prevent Illness (cont.)	Restore Health (cont.)
England	Take cod liver oil daily.	Get lots of fresh air. Wrap up warmly. Drink brown ale after cleaning a sick room to prevent catching the disease.	Fever: Drink mint or chamomile tea. Cough and congestion: Put formaldehyde crystals in a plastic bag and place on the chest. Mumps: Apply hot mustard poultice. Nosebleed: Put a cold key down your back. General illness: Feed bread cubes in warm sweet milk (pobs).
Ethiopia	Make sure food is on the table for everyone.	Give people water blessed by the spirit (church) to drink.	Pray.
France	Eat a big lunch with different foods. Drink drinks with herbs. Drink soup. Eat chocolate. Take cod liver oil. Eat bread and butter. Put hot stones under the bed. Put iron nails in water.	Take cod liver oil (oil of fish liver).	General illness: Drink *Daliborng* water. Cuts and bruises: Put castor oil on right away to prevent pain and swelling.

Nation (cont.)	Maintain Health (cont.)	Protect Health or Prevent Illness (cont.)	Restore Health (cont.)
Germany	Eat meatball soup, lots of vegetables, and good food. Every day before going to bed eat an apple. Take cod liver oil. Get fresh air, and work hard.	Take castor oil daily. Dress warmly. Wrap salted herring and wear it around your neck. Drink boneset tea daily.	Colds: Apply mustard plaster. Visit neighborhood pow-wow doctors. Worms: Eat hot garlic milk with honey. Any illness: Eat chicken soup. Cold: Place a cut onion next to your bed while sleeping to help breathing.
Greece	Eat good food. Drink chamomile tea. Wear a wool undershirt. Never go out of house after bath.	Eat 1 tablespoon of honey each day during the cold months to prevent colds. Keep warm. Wear amulets containing flowers from the Epitafio on Holy Friday. Pray to God.	Stomach ailments: Drink mountain tea (mint tea with honey). Pray. Colds and pneumonia: Use cupping (cotton inserted in a glass and lit with a match and left on the back). Earaches: Warm olive oil and place it in the ear.
Haiti	Eat well. Eat fresh foods.	Drink tea every day made with sorosi to increase appetite.	Fever: Mix castor oil, alcohol, and shallot. Heat the mixture, rub together in hand, and rub all over the body.

SELECTED HEALTH TRADITIONS (CONT.)

Nation (cont.)	Maintain Health (cont.)	Protect Health or Prevent Illness (cont.)	Restore Health (cont.)
India	Eat vegetables. Eat healthy foods and exercise.	Use black pepper and licorice.	Indigestion: Drink cumin water. Upset stomach: Drink buttermilk and fenugreek. Sore throat: Drink turmeric in hot milk.
Ireland	Eat lots of potatoes and cabbage. Wear warm clothing. Keep clean. Get fresh air, and work hard. Sleep with the window open a crack.	In spring time take nettles (wild), boil them down, and then drink it. Eat porridge at night before going to bed. Pray. Do not go to bed with wet hair. Drink nettle soup to clear the blood. Put camphor on a cloth and wear around neck.	Drink plenty of tea and Guiness (ale). Cold: Eat a whole raw onion and have a shot of whiskey. "Wind," (flatulance): Face rearend to the fire. Boils and cuts: Wrap hot bread, sugar, soap in linen cloth and place it on the wound to prevent infection. Cold or flu: Apply poultices and molasses. Fever: Tie onions to wrists or dirty sock around the neck.

SELECTED HEALTH TRADITIONS (CONT.)

Nation (cont.)	Maintain Health (cont.)	Protect Health or Prevent Illness (cont.)	Restore Health (cont.)
Italy	Love each other. Eat chicken soup. Wear and eat garlic. Drink a glass of wine a day. Wear a camphor bag around the neck. Eat fresh fruit and vegetables every day. Get lots of sleep.	Children should wear a pouch with raw garlic around neck to keep unhealthy children away. "Spring cleaning:" Drink bitter greens boiled in water.	Cold and cough: Put warm to hot red brick wrapped in wool cloth on chest. Inhale very hot water with turpentine, or drink boiled wine with apples. Get rid of the evil eye or to cast out any evil spirits: Drink cod liver oil. Colic: Drink fennel seed tea. Pray to God. Upset stomach: Drink water mixed with sugar and bay leaf.
Jamaica	Eat a lot of tropical fruits, especially mangoes. Get a lot of exercise in the form of chores. Take weekly cathartics to wash out the system and drink cerasee tea (each Sunday).	Drink different kinds of herb and bush teas. Get plenty of rest. Drink whole milk and beef soup, and eat fresh fruit and vegetables.	Take medicine in the form of herbal bushes. Pray to the Lord for help. Back pain: Use a poultice. Stomach problems: Drink dandelion and ginger tea.

SELECTED HEALTH TRADITIONS (CONT.)

Nation (cont.)	Maintain Health (cont.)	Protect Health or Prevent Illness (cont.)	Restore Health (cont.)
Japan	Children: Every morning (even in winter) massage his or her naked body to keep healthy.	Gargle with salt water. Sleep well, eat good things, and exercise.	Keep body warm with blanket and sleep. Cure asthma attacks: *yaeto* usually burned on upper back and shoulders. Upset stomach: Drink green tea.
Lithuania	Eat fresh fruits and vegetables. Take herbal enemas.	Eat good food, get plenty of rest.	Apply mustard plasters. Colds and stomach aches: Drink brandy.
Mexico	Eat eggs and bread. Sleep and drink tea.	Use herbs and amulets.	Use herbs, and visit traditional healers.
Netherlands	Practice cleanliness. Eat pancakes. Eat cooked vegetables.	Make sure to get up on the right foot. Eat a lot of fruit. Eat chicken soup.	Headache: Mop the floor with ammonia. Eat soft-boiled eggs.
Norway	Eat fruit and vegetables.	Wear coats and pants.	Eat soup and drink hot chocolate.
Pakistan	Take lemon in summer to beat the heat. Eat chicken soup in the winter.	Eat garlic to prevent colds in the winter.	Headache: Drink green tea. Gas in stomach: Drink ginger.

SELECTED HEALTH TRADITIONS (CONT.)

Nation (cont.)	Maintain Health (cont.)	Protect Health or Prevent Illness (cont.)	Restore Health (cont.)
Philippines	Pray. Eat healthy food, such as vegetables, meat, chicken, and fruits and have excellent hygiene.	Eat pigeon soup. After working in the fields, soak feet in salted water. Avoid too much sun or rain.	Eat chicken soup. Painful joints: Pound ginger mix with coconut oil and massage. Stomach ache: Toast uncooked rice until brown, add water, mix and drink the fluid. Wounds: Boil guava leaves and drink the fluid, or grind guava leaves and apply to the wound to cure fresh wound faster. Take herbal medicines.
Poland	Eat chicken soup. Tie garlic around neck. Eat well (fat). Drink tea with honey or cinnamon. Drink tea from Camile tree flowers. Practice cleanliness.	Dress warmly. Eat broth. Use herbal tonics. Eat garlic.	Practice blood letting using leeches. Colds: Eat chicken soup, drink hot tea, apply mustard plasters, hot cups, compresses; drink raspberry juice. Stomach problems: Drink mint tea.

SELECTED HEALTH TRADITIONS (CONT.)

Nation (cont.)	Maintain Health (cont.)	Protect Health or Prevent Illness (cont.)	Restore Health (cont.)
Prussia	Drink herbal teas. Eat plantain leaves. Drink tea with honey and ground ambgor everyday. Use feverfew and mint.	Wear Yiddish amulets and keep good luck coins.	To draw out infection: Apply pitch from pine trees.
Romania	Saturday night bath for all children in the same water. Eat a balanced diet. Eat chicken soup. Eat mush and drink fresh milk.	Eat garlic daily.	Cold or flu: Eat chicken soup. To purify blood: Eat garlic. Constipation: Eat yogurt and herbs. Warts: Apply poultice of chicken skin and mustard.
Russia	Eat chicken soup. Keep warm. Eat lots of vegetables. Take cod liver oil. Eat raw garlic and onions.	Wear garlic bags around the neck. Children wear camphor enclosed in a cloth necklace. Wear dry socks. Keep the feet warm and the head covered.	Colds and flu: Use cupping. Colds and sore throat: Drink milk with butter; or apply a mustard plaster using dry mustard in a gauze bag and dipping into water and placing on chest.

SELECTED HEALTH TRADITIONS (CONT.)

Nation (cont.)	Maintain Health (cont.)	Protect Health or Prevent Illness (cont.)	Restore Health (cont.)
Russia (cont.)			Sore throat: Drink *guggle muggle* (a drink of hot milk, honey [or sugar] and butter) or boil together 1 jigger of wine or brandy, juice of 1 lemon and 1 tbs. of honey. Drink. Stye: Rub eye with wedding ring and spit three times.
Slovakia	Eat chicken soup. Wash hands. Eat cabbage soup. Eat prune desserts to keep in balance. Eat garlic and sauerkraut (also juice from it) especially in winter. Drink herbal teas (chamomile for general health).	Get lots of sleep and exercise. Eat garlic. Get fresh air. Eat a lot of vegetables. Keep dry and warm.	Cold: Drink tea with honey and lemon. Pray (novenas—nine days of praying). Infections: Epsom salts in bath water. Sore throat: Drink hot milk with squeezed garlic in it plus 2 teaspoons of honey. Heavy cough, pain in chest: Heat fat in a small pot, apply to a cloth and put on chest until it is covered with a sight film of fat. Cover with plastic (to keep it warm) and blend into towel and try to sleep with it overnight. Indigestion: Eat garlic soup.

SELECTED HEALTH TRADITIONS (CONT.)

Nation (cont.)	Maintain Health (cont.)	Protect Health or Prevent Illness (cont.)	Restore Health (cont.)
Thailand	Take care of children.	Eat healthy foods.	Use herbs, plants.
Turkey	Eat a cup of yogurt a day.	Drink hot milk with egg yolk and sugar. Keep your feet warm and head cool. Don't worry too much.	Insect bites: Cover with mud mixed with urine. Sprains: Apply garlic and raisin poultice to the area. Toothache: Drink brandy. Minor illness: Boil mint with lemon and drink. Common cold: Drink linden flower tea. Blunt injuries (minor): Cover with dough and hammered meat. Stye: Apply garlic.
Ukraine	Eat chicken soup. Drink vodka.	Eat healthy food. Bundle up in cold weather. Drink vodka.	Coughs: Use cupping. Fever: Apply mustard packs. Constipation: Use enemas. Cold (stuffy nose): Wrap boiled potatoes in a towel, hold on nose, also mix honey and water as nose drops. Drink vodka.

SELECTED HEALTH TRADITIONS (CONT.)

Nation (cont.)	Maintain Health (cont.)	Protect Health or Prevent Illness (cont.)	Restore Health (cont.)
Venezuela		Use homeopathic medicine.	Upset stomach: Drink hot milk with butter.
Vietnam	Eat well. Eat soup and drink tea.	Use massage. Take steambaths. Apply tiger oil.	Use Chinese medicine.

From: Spector, R., Rutberg, C., and Byron, E. Data collected from visitors to "Immigrant Health Traditions" Exhibit, Ellis Island Immigration Museum, May, 1994–January, 1995.

Cross-Cultural
Health-Care Guide*

The following guidelines will help you understand your clients better and allow you to provide them with the help they need.

Preparing
- Understand your own cultural values and biases.
- Acquire basic knowledge of cultural values, health beliefs and practices for the client groups you serve.
- Be respectful of, interested in, and understanding of other cultures without being judgmental.

Enhancing Communication
- Determine the client's level of fluency in English and arrange for an interpreter, if needed.
- Ask how the client prefers to be addressed.
- Allow the client to choose seating for comfortable personal space and eye contact.

*From: (Adapted for nursing) Schilling, B. and Brannon, E. *Cross-Cultural Counseling—A Guide for Nutrition and Health Counselors.* Alexandria, VA: (United States Department of Agriculture, United States Department of Health and Human Services, Nutrition and Technical Services Division, September, 1986), p. 19. Reprinted with permission.

- Avoid body language that may be offensive or misunderstood.
- Speak directly to the client, whether an interpreter is present or not.
- Choose a speech rate and style that promotes understanding and demonstrates respect for the client.
- Avoid slang, technical jargon, and complex sentences.
- Use open-ended questions or questions phrased in several ways to obtain information.
- Determine the client's reading ability before using written materials in the teaching process.

Promoting Positive Change

- Build on cultural practices, reinforcing those that are positive, and promoting change only in those that are harmful.
- Check for client understanding and acceptance of recommendations.
- *Remember:* Not all seeds of knowledge fall into a fertile environment to produce change. Of those that do, some will take years to germinate. Be patient and provide nursing in a culturally appropriate environment to promote positive health behavior.

SAMPLE GRID FOR CULTURAL HEALTH ASSESSMENT

	Physical	Mental	Spiritual
Maintain Health			
Protect Health			
Restore Health			

SAMPLE GRID FOR CULTURAL HEALTH ASSESSMENT

	Physical	Mental	Spiritual
Maintain Health			
Protect Health			
Restore Health			

SAMPLE GRID FOR CULTURAL HEALTH ASSESSMENT

	Physical	Mental	Spiritual
Maintain Health			
Protect Health			
Restore Health			

Notes

Notes

Notes

Notes

Notes